ACKNOWLEDGEMENT

I sincerely acknowledge the help of these colleagues and friends, who reviewed and offered excellent suggestions for parts or all of this manuscript.

Stanley Cohen, B.S., M.Ed. Ed.D
Executive Vice Dean for Educational Support
Health Professions Division, Nova
Southeastern University

Neil A. Natkow, A.B., DO
Distinguished Faculty
College of Osteopathic Medicine
Nova Southeastern University

Sandy D. Melnick, B.A., M.D. (my son)
Medical Director
Acute Partial Care Program
Atlantic Care Regional Medical Center

DEDICATION

I dedicate this book
to the memory of my late wife

ANITA

whom I still love dearly

OTHER BOOKS BY THE AUTHOR

*Pediatrics: Some Uncommon Views on Some
Common Problems*

*Professionally Speaking: Public Speaking for Health
Professionals*

*Oratorio Para Profesionales de la Salud
(Professionally Speaking)*

*Medical Writing 101: A Primer for Health
Professionals*

Parenthood: Laugh and Understand Your Child

Ethical Problems in Pediatrics: A Dozen Dilemmas

*Effective Medical Communication
An Anthology of Columns from The DO Magazine*

Looking Back . . . at SECOM

Practicing for Practice

*Melnick on Writing
An Anthology of Columns from the American Medical Writers Association*

*Osteopathic Tales
Stories tracing one DO's travel along the path of the Osteopathic Profession
from Rejection and Discrimination to Recognition and Acceptance*

Giving Your Child Medication . . . Safely

MONOGRAPHS

So you've been asked to speak...

*Sandy, We Love You
(with Anita Melnick)*

Who Will I Tell?

Nothing is Risk-Free in Health Care

A Handbook for Patients

Arnold Melnick,
DO, MSc, DHL (Hon), FACOP

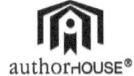
authorHOUSE®

AuthorHouse™ LLC
1663 Liberty Drive
Bloomington, IN 47403
www.authorhouse.com
Phone: 1-800-839-8640

Published by AuthorHouse 06/25/2014

ISBN: 978-1-4969-2249-6 (sc)
ISBN: 978-1-4969-2250-2 (e)

Library of Congress Control Number: 2014911707

TABLE OF CONTENTS

PREFACE

First, a cardinal principle that affects everything in all our lives: THERE IS ALMOST NOTHING IN LIFE THAT IS FREE OF RISK!

Just think of flying in airplanes, travelling in an automobile, eating food (especially from strange or unknown sources), riding a Ferris wheel in an amusement park — and almost anything else you can imagine. And if that's hard to believe, ask why all of the operators/owners involved with them carry heavy insurance.

Thus, the title of this book is *Nothing Is Risk-Free in Health Care.* It is not a "scare" book. It is not meant to frighten patients about their health care. It is not any indictment of medical care workers or institutions. Here we speak of risks for errors— and mostly they are accidental. Yes, once a year or so we may read of some criminal activity involving health, but here, we will talk about health or safety errors — mistakes, blunders, lapses, not deliberately harmful actions. Fortunately, almost everyone and everything in healthcare occurs with caring and dedicated intent— but accidents (errors) do happen.

What is this book, then? It is a compilation of widely accepted information about risks, both common and rare, in the field of health care. Committees and boards have been set up all around the country — the Food and Drug Administration, United States Pharmacopeia and many medical societies, for example— whose sole purpose is to study and make recommendations to reduce these risks. And some progress has already occurred.

Among the key reports in this field was the first major one, issued in 1998 by the Institute of Medicine, a prestigious organization. It was a ground-breaking report titled *To Err is Human: Building a Safer Health System* and was followed closely by *Crossing the Quality Chasm.* Both strongly reviewed the healthcare system and started a widespread movement to create greater patient safety in the United States.

The federal Agency for Healthcare Research and Quality (AHRQ) issued in 2001 its report *Making Health Care Safer: A Critical Analysis of Patient Safety Practices.* Just recently (2013), the AHRQ published a follow-up *Making Health Care Safer II: An Updated Critical Analysis of the Evidence for Patient Safety Practices.* It listed 41 patient safety strategies and encouraged adoption of the top ten, all directed at preventing, among other things, medication errors, bedsores and healthcare-associated infections.

All these efforts from the Institute of Medicine, from agencies of the federal government and from other groups is overwhelming evidence that there is much risk in our health care system. And it empathizes the need for further study, new changes, and careful attention by patients and health care personnel.

Why then is this book being written?

This book is written purely to alert patients (and their families) to some of these risks, to familiarize them with the dangers as much as we can and to offer suggestions for trying to avoid them or minimize them.

But the one suggestion, above all, is

**YOU MUST TAKE RESPONSIBILITY
FOR YOUR OWN HEALTH CARE!**

CHAPTER ONE

A Look at the Dangers

Sunshine is good for you. Water is good for you. The sun provides Vitamin D, and water is essential to life. But over-used, under-used or misused, both can be most harmful. Everything in our lives that relates to health falls into the same category. Nothing is risk-free – we must constantly be aware of the truth of this maxim. We must learn to use everything with caution, even though any particular item, used properly, may be beneficial for the most part.

Those of us living in the 21st century are most fortunate: medicine, medical science, pharmaceutical research and all their associated fields, have provided us with care and help unsurpassed in the history of man. We live longer lives, we are physically stronger, we have less illness. In addition, we now have visions and glimpses of things to come that will improve even today's wonderful health aids: atomic possibilities, stem cell possibilities, genetic research, robotic surgery, and many others.

However, being surrounded by these magnificent health aids does not eliminate the need for us to be wary and alert.

We must examine them, understand their value and be knowledgeable of the potentially harmful effects—in order to protect ourselves even further. That is the purpose of this book.

Every prescription comes from the pharmacy with a formally-printed list of side effects, things for which we must be watchful. We are all familiar with these inserts. First, they are there because the FDA requires it. Why? — especially since most of these side effects are relatively rare? So that you will be alerted to them, and can avoid difficulties later. However, there are no lists available about physicians, hospitals, health insurers, third-party payers, and the myriad of other health advantages we are fortunate to have. Even health "literature", such as print advertising and television commercials, carry warnings of dangers and side-effects of medications they advertise (by federal law, they must do so because it is so important). Warning: this book does not point fingers at any of those institutions or at the people involved. There are very, very few, actually infinitesimal numbers of persons in the health care field who deliberately set out to do harm (these few are really criminals but unfortunately they do exist). And, fortunately, there are only a few whose sloppiness and disregard may lead to problems. All people engaged in the health field, professional and lay, are human beings first—errors occur, problems arise, and sometimes dire consequences result. Nothing in this book is meant to cast blame or to indict anyone.

My only aim is to call attention to problems that can affect us all and to offer some guidelines on how we can perhaps help ourselves. Somehow, all of us must personally become aware of our potential "bumps in the road" for us and always be on the lookout for them. No matter how low the percentage of bad effects — and the percentage is very low — just one is too many. This, too, is the purpose of this book.

The Agency for Healthcare Research and Quality of the U.S. Department of Health and Human Services has said it succinctly: "Medical errors can occur anywhere in the health care system: in hospitals, clinics, surgery centers, doctors' offices, nursing homes, pharmacies and patients' homes. Errors can involve medication, surgery, diagnosis, equipment or laboratory reports." And so often, errors involve more than one source.

Because of the nature of this subject, there are many cross-overs of material—for example, some things refer to physicians as well as pharmacists, some refer to hospitals as well as physicians. Similarly, with other areas, I have tried to put the information under the most logical and convenient chapter headings; there is some unavoidable duplication.

In this book, practitioner refers to any one-on-one health person, including physicians, dentists, medical specialists, nurse practitioners, physician assistants, optometrists and podiatrists plus the so-called secondary health individuals, such as nurses, therapists, technicians, etc. All are trusted professionals and each field has its own area of expertise.

While there are thousands of instances of risks becoming real, and causing great difficulty, when compared to the millions of patients receiving care, millions undergoing surgery, millions being admitted to hospitals and perhaps billions taking prescriptions, the actual incidence is small. However, if you or a loved one is one of that small number, the incidence for you is 100%. So the risk is always there and must be kept in mind in all medical care situations.

And now, to the Conclusions.

CHAPTER TWO

Conclusions

(Unlike most treatises, I shall present my conclusions first, so that you know where we—you and I—are going. Then I shall develop the themes pertaining to those conclusions, so that you will understand how they developed and why they are important.)

1. (The Cardinal Principle) All of us are responsible for our own individual care and, obviously, we are responsible for our young children's care and sometimes our older or incapacitated parents. That means:

2. Remember that you are the paying customer. You are not a beggar. You (or someone on your behalf) is paying for the services you seek and receive. You must see that those services are rendered—in a kind and caring way.

3. Since you are the buyer, it must be *caveat emptor,* buyer beware. Ask questions until you understand —understand what is being done, how it is being

done and why it is being done. You are entitled to proper care but just as important, you are entitled to a full understanding.

4. You must be aware of the resources available to you in those few instances in which services do not meet reasonable expectations.

5. **YOU MUST TAKE RESPONSIBILITY FOR YOUR OWN HEALTH CARE**

CHAPTER THREE

Physicians and other Practitioners

With all the wonderful advances that have come to the medical world, there have been a number of significant changes in medical care. As an example, there are no such things as physician house calls today. No longer does (or can) a physician call at the patient's home to minister to him when he is sick – except for a recent revival of this kind of care for some of our confined elders and the development of some practices that are confined solely to house calls. The old classic picture of the physician sitting by the bed of a desperately ill patient is an anachronism today. It represents a time when just sitting by the bed was about the only thing a doctor could do.

A number of the old amenities have gone by the board—brought on by two things: great advances in medicine (for example, antibiotics abolishing the need for sitting by the patient as he or she goes through the storm of a violent infection) and the totally changed economics of practice (for example, insurance or influence of third-party payers).

Physicians today do not have sufficient time needed to take an unhurried history, talk leisurely with the patient during the physical examination, tell the patient the diagnosis and explain what the treatment will be, including what the prescriptions are and what they are for. Recently, it was estimated that the average pediatric visit was 14.5 minutes long. Other estimates put adult visits at an average of 11 minutes. Occasionally, visits need only be that short, especially a brief re-visit, a follow-up or a reporting of lab work to the patient. Certainly, that is not sufficient time for first visit or for a difficult case. There must be enough time to ensure good care. Matters of time insufficiency often come about because of the pressures of practice, insurance pressures, HMO requirements (insistence on seeing a certain number of patients each hour), and in some rare situations, the physician's decision.

More typical today is the patient's filling in a questionnaire in the waiting room (medical history, as well as financial information). Usually today it is in the reverse order — (financial first), sitting (for a variable time) in a waiting room, sitting in an examination room (a few to many minutes later), seeing the doctor, getting a brief-to-complete examination (depending on the doctor and the complaint), getting the physician's diagnosis—and sometimes not, and getting instructions or prescriptions (sometimes from the doctor and sometimes from an office staff member—often not a nurse or other professional).

Choosing a Physician

For the benefit of your medical care, you should choose a physician or appropriate health professional whom others think is highly capable of helping you. When searching for a new health professional, inquire of trusted friends, neighbors, relatives, co-workers or a health professional that you have used in a different field (even this system is not fool-proof, but it helps). Your physician should be competent (as most are) and, almost as important, you and he/she should be compatible and able to communicate satisfactorily.

There is not much value in choosing a competent doctor, then not being able to get the information you should, or not feeling comfortable in his/her office or not having full confidence in that doctor's ability. I feel that most practitioners would not want you to have these feelings. Of course, most patients cannot accurately evaluate a doctor's medical competence, or measure it for varying medical conditions, but you should feel that by and large the practitioner is good enough to be your doctor. And that you don't dread going into his/her office.

Your obligations

After choosing a physician for yourself or your family, you have certain obligations and responsibilities to ensure that your care is the best by:

- Paying attention to everything that is said and done in the physician's office. It is not unusual that patients, under the stress of being examined and worrying about a diagnosis or therapy, will not remember everything they are told. Most of the time, it is wise to have a spouse, another family member or close friend to accompany you. Together there is a higher chance that the most important things will be recalled.

- Asking as many questions as needed to understand what is going on. Don't stop until your questions are satisfactorily answered.

- Not leaving without being told the diagnosis (or what you are being treated for, or what you are being studied or tested for).

- Knowing what medication the doctor is prescribing, how it is to be used and what it is specifically for – and possible side effects or dangers.

- Looking at a prescription handed to you by other than the physician, to see that it matches what the doctor has told you. And if you are not sure, ask and ask again.

- Understanding what follow-up is suggested: re-visit, consultation, laboratory studies – who, what, when, where, and why?

- Not leaving the office until you get all the needed information.

- Making inquiries politely — not rudely or challengingly.

- Asking questions, not making accusations.

Some patients feel that this is imposing on the doctor's time. It is not. He/she owes you this. You or someone — insurance company, HMO, or even governments (or a social service agency in the case of indigent patients) is compensating the physician, so you are entitled to full care.

Perhaps you could speed things up on your visit to the doctor if you prepared a list of your symptoms (complaints), in the order of how they affect you. Do this before you leave home for the doctor's office— just brief notes as reminder to yourself.

These may seem overwhelming or time-consuming, but actually take only a small amount of concentration and a only a brief moment or two, and in the long run they will also save your doctor's time. If your practitioner refuses to co-operate for this minimal information (and fortunately there are only a few of these), it's time to seek another doctor. And since it is your life, and your money, and your time, you have every right to seek a new doctor if you are not happy, for whatever reason. Your doctor owes you this information. Similarly, a doctor has the legal right to dismiss a patient (for whatever reason) as long as the physician does not abandon the patient.

Medical Errors

Medical errors may involve physicians, other practitioners, medication, hospitals or any other portion of the health care system. Often errors are a combination of these.

Examples are plentiful, but a few specific ones must be worthwhile mentioning. I am not pointing them out as extreme examples or common examples, but just examples. Readers may recall that in the spring of 2003, a teenager at Duke University Medical center was given a heart-lung transplant (you know it must be a major institution if they do this kind of surgery). He needed a blood transfusion. The donor was of a wrong blood type. Apparently nobody checked to be sure that the blood type matched the patient's. The youngster had a severe reaction with rejection of the transplant. Even with immediate remedial action and another transplant, the teenager died. Many fingers could be pointed in this case, and probably have been.

Another interesting case recently was the young lady subjected to a double mastectomy after a positive report for cancer. Two days after the surgery, it was discovered that the positive cancer test belonged to a different patient, and this patient was actually cancer-free. Medical errors, according to the Institute of Medicine, cause or contribute to more than one million injuries and illnesses each year.

In one instance, a child received 10 times the calculated dose of Coumadin (a blood thinner) for his age in an error probably due to a misplaced decimal point. Misplaced decimal points, along with incorrect weight conversions and wrong selection of medication seem to be among the leading mistakes in prescribing for children. As an indication, The Royal Hospital for Sick Children in Glasgow surveyed their records and found 1 error for every 682 pediatric admissions.

The National Institute of Medicine has estimated that there are 400,000 drug-related injuries every year.

All of these are rare instances but it is important to keep mind always that such exigencies — always unexpected — do occur.

Common Risks in the Physician's Office

UNDERSTAND THIS: While possible risks are listed here, remember that most doctors are caring and competent, and all have their own personalities – and idiosyncrasies. That means that the practitioner's style of practice and his or her personality will vary from doctor to doctor. Examples: some will talk more and some will talk less. Some will be warmer or more informal personalities, some will be more formal. Some may order batteries of tests and some may depend on their clinical ability and knowledge. Whether your physician orders many tests or no tests at all is no indication of his or her competence. Informing you of such risks is not an indictment of anyone. For example, even though all poisonous substances you may buy in a store have directions on the container telling what to do if the substance is accidentally ingested, the number of times that happens is infinitesimal, BUT THE RISK ALWAYS NEEDS TO BE PRESENTED—so that you will be aware of potential risks.

Some risks:

1. Not getting an appointment soon enough when an acute situation arises (either first visit or on re-appointment). No one can accurately set standard or uniform times for setting appointments, but they should be reasonable. A patient with severe chest pain cannot wait two days for an appointment On the other hand, chronic low back pain is probably one that might have to wait for a routine appointment. I know of several instances in which a patient calls the physician's office and is greeted with "Will you hold the phone, please?" and then with a click, the receptionist not even waiting to see whether this is an urgent or emergency call. In those offices, a better system is needed. In some instances recently, the initial phone message is something like, "If this is an emergency, go immediately to

the nearest hospital emergency room." A notable improvement!

2. The physician who is so busy all the time so that you have to sit in the waiting room for more than 30 minutes every time you go. Yes, it is possible to conduct a practice so that, most of the time, the waits are minimal. Yes, emergencies arise, but after a few months of practice the office should be able to estimate time schedules most of the time. Doctors may over-book deliberately for many reasons, some because they are plagued with "no-shows" throwing the office way off schedule, some so that there are always patients waiting in the office, and even a few to impress other patients with how busy they are. This renders a disservice to you, to the other patients and even to the physician.

3. Kept unclothed in an examining room for inordinate periods of time—really just another waiting room, but this one you cannot escape from. If this happens frequently, register your unhappiness with the physician directly and politely—not the office staff. There is no justification for this happening frequently.

4. Hurried (and harried) time with the physician, making you feel that you are imposing on the practitioner's time or you think you are not getting an adequate examination or diagnostic opinion. Speak up!

5. A physician who tolerates no discussion of your case or pooh-poohs any concerns or questions you raise about the diagnosis or treatment.

An extreme example of this happened to a friend. He is a lawyer with considerable medical knowledge. He went to visit a dermatologist for the first time. As he sat on the examining table, the doctor came in and walked over to him, and reached out immediately for his arm to examine the affected skin area. Softly, the patient asked, "Aren't you going to wash your hands first?" — invoking a serious medical procedure. With anger on his face, the dermatologist blurted out, "Get out of my office. I don't want you for a patient" and stormed out. If he had washed them in another room, he should have said so. If he forgot (or consistently did this) he might have apologized and washed his hands in front of the patient, establishing a connection with the patient. Of course, my lawyer-friend left right away and went to another physician.

6. Rudeness on the part of the doctor or his staff or both. Rudeness by office staff, in person or by telephone, should be reported to your physician –he/she doesn't want that in the office any more than you do. If the physician is rude, it usually will suggest a rude staff—seek another office.

7. Incorrect diagnosis or treatment can occur in any situation. No doctor will claim to be infallible and no mistakes are made deliberately. If any part of your visit, especially diagnosis or treatment, seems questionable or suspicious, you should seriously talk to the doctor immediately and be sure you are satisfied with the answers.

8. Failure to recommend consultation when the problem seems to require one.

Here's an example of an unclassifiable risk. My wife was hospitalized with a complaint of difficulty walking and some memory defect. The orthopedic surgeon who was called in consultation, and apparently didn't read her chart before seeing her, went into her room and asked her if she could show him how she walked. Getting out of bed, she took one step and fell on the floor, fracturing her arm. Perhaps if he had read the chart as he should have before examining the patient, this accident would not have happened. Another kind of error! (Note: he also billed her for casting the arm— at his regular rate.)

Other "risks": Annoying, but less interfering

Think of this: You go into the food market. Each time, the clerk is snooty and rude. That does not diminish the quality of the food you are buying or change the price or interfere in any way with that purchase. So you have several choices. Next time, go to a different market (if it carries the same product). Or keep going back because that product is so dear to you that you are willing to put up with a little annoyance to obtain it. Or call the clerk's rudeness to someone (his manager, the company, or to the clerk himself; he may not be aware he is doing it).

Similar situations can occur in visiting a health practitioner. Little things arise that that are "risks" in that office – BUT the quality of care may not be at all affected. You have the same choices.

My colleague, Stanley Cohen, EdD, psychologist and educator who teaches medical ethics to health professions students, did a survey of patients and compiled a list of frequent complaints. He shared them with me. Over a large number of people, the reoccurrence of these complaints establishes that they are significant in the eyes of patients. I will add my personal comments to each one.

I feel my doctor is always in a hurry and I never have enough time

It is true that doctors are frequently rushed—extra time consumed with an unexpected patient problem, delay is getting out of the hospital, over-scheduling, and many other reasons. When it is persistent, you have a good reason to feel uncomfortable; there could be better time management in the physician's office. You have the same choices described above.

One of the best approaches for the problem is: at the start of your next visit, to say to the physician (quietly, softly and without anger), "Dr. Jones, I have something to tell you before you begin. Every time I come here I feel rushed, that you are in a hurry and that I never get enough time. Is there something we can do about that? I don't want to feel uncomfortable coming in here, and I want to still continue to have you as my physician." His or her response will then guide you further. Then it's your decision.

The perception of time in a visit is often different between patient and doctor. One internist I know always sits down before starting to talk with his patients—that gives the patient a perception that he is not rushing and intends to spend whatever time is needed.

One of my old medical school professors (a surgeon), once told us, as a teaching parable, that if you have only 20 seconds to visit with a hospitalized patient, go in the room, sit on the side of the bed, take the patient's hand and spend the 20 seconds talking to and listening to him/her.

When I'm in the doctor's office, I always have to wait a long time

Your approach should be similar to the problem above. Talk to the doctor before he starts your next visit. Explain what is bothering you, and ask whether there is some way to solve the problem. Be firm. Prepare what you are going to say so that it is brief and concise but do not become belligerent. Anger often begets anger.

If you cannot resolve the problem with him—if his reasons are unacceptable ("I'm a busy doctor", "I have a lot of patients to see", "You see how many patients want to see me; there's nothing I can do" or the doctor gets angry with you), your choice is to seek another doctor (and, for the most part, there are plenty of good physicians out there) or to decide that the doctor is important enough to you that you are willing to put up with the inconveniences and won't get upset about it again.

I feel intimidated. Are my concerns important enough to take up the valuable time of the doctor?

Intimidation is a feeling that comes from within us; if you don't want to be intimidated, you won't be. Unless the physician is a bully (and I think there are very few of these around) or so overbearing or impressed with his own importance (some doctors fit this but they also occur in all occupations), the problem is you. Sure, the doctor is busy, but he is there to serve you. Someone is paying him to serve you and you are entitled to reasonable attention. So you should not be intimidated. You are important and your concerns are important—and most doctors will pay attention.

There are exceptions. I think of the physician – a family doctor—who set a timer on his desk for five minutes every time a patient came in. He would say, "You have five minutes. You can use it to talk or for me to examine you." Besides this being arrogant, I don't know how a physician can give adequate service to any patient – take a history, do a physical examination or provide treatment (even write a prescription)—in five minutes.

Don't be intimidated. Exert your rights. If you meet resistance, change doctors.

How do I encourage my doctor to hear me and listen to what I have to say?

Some surveys have shown that, when a patient presents a complaint, doctors on average listen for only 11 seconds before interrupting and interpreting. Insufficient time! Your physician should give you a reasonable time to explain what is bothering you, then he will ask questions, then examine you. I believe that most physicians do this, but if they happen to be rushing, it will seem to the patient like only 11 seconds.

But there is a precaution for the patient. First, do not take up the doctor's time with irrelevant chatter: "How's your wife? Did you get your car fixed? Isn't it terrible what happed to the governor?" That wastes everyone's time. Most important, be prepared: think long about your problem and be so organized that you will not stumble and will not need long times to think about answers to questions. Write down your concerns ahead of time.

Simple answers can be prepared. Think about why you are going the doctor, so that you can answer quickly. Not just, "I have a cough" but know when it started, how bad it is, what bothers you most about it, whether it is accompanied by any other complaint or symptom, what makes it worse, what makes it better—the same information you might share with a friend when talking about mutual complaints. That will save a lot of time in the doctor's office and, if the problem is you, this will speed things up. We make lists when we go to the market, so we won't forget. If we have an electrical problem in our homes, we call an electrician and make a list of the problems and their complications so we won't leave anything out.

What should I do if I am interrupted?

Answer: the same as you would do if anyone interrupted you. Try these, depending on circumstances: "Just a minute, doctor, I'm not finished," or "Please hear me out," or "I have one more important thing to add." Again, this should be done politely and without anger or rancor.

I don't know enough to ask questions. I don't know what to ask. I feel that my questions are stupid.

For the most part, the important questions are: What is my diagnosis? What does that mean? What is the outlook for my condition? What is that laboratory work (or x-ray) for? What did it tell you? What is the treatment you are prescribing? These will cover most situations.

If you are still unsatisfied with the answer—or dissatisfied—try something like, "Doctor, what questions should I be asking you after what you just said?" It's your visit, so don't be afraid to ask.

Questions about your health are never stupid, or should not be considered stupid by medical personnel. If you knew what to ask and knew exactly how to phrase the question and really knew the answers before you asked, you obviously wouldn't ask the question. Ask! Ask!

My doctor looks at the chart and not at me.

The reasons for this are myriad. It may lie in the doctor's personality or his rushing or whatever. Patients with an embarrassing condition or complaint might even prefer for the doctor not to look. Charts are important in these days of third-party medicine and the malpractice environment. Perhaps your doctor wants to be sure that he gets all the information correctly—or he is scanning your record for connections with what you are telling him.

This occurrence is somewhat complicated by the advent of computers, with physicians who utilize the computer for more efficient history taking with greater accuracy. It may be something we have to bear with until something better comes along.

If you are uncomfortable with his not looking at you, call it to his attention —nicely. I'm sure he will respond. Or you can ask questions to elicit the information you are seeking.

My doctor doesn't seem to take me seriously.

This is not a common happening. Perhaps it is something the patient has said or done. Ask your doctor why. If he's fair, he will tell you. Then work it out together, as you would with a spouse. Both of you are concerned that you get the proper health care.

My doctor says, "At your age . . ."

If your doctor says that without a thorough evaluation, run to the nearest physician who cares for older folks. Attributing an elder's complaints to age without a thorough investigation is poor geriatric care, and usually is an evasion. Age cannot be blamed for most complaints but sometimes if there are no diagnostic findings, it may be. Example: if you have joint pains, it could be arthritis—and, yes, that often is a disease of older folks. But before the doctor can say definitely it is arthritis and that it is the arthritis of aging as opposed to other types of arthritis, he must go through whatever diagnostic procedures that are necessary. Then, it is not "At your age . . ." but rather "You have arthritis, which is common at your age but there are things we can do to help you."

Just because a patient is older is not a reason to minimize his problems or treat him as though he must accept problems in old age. There are many healthy older people.

The office staff is not always helpful or courteous

The faults here may be either that the staff is mimicking the behavior of the physician, who also does not seem to extend help or courtesy to the patient. Or, perhaps the doctor does not observe or supervise the staff closely enough to know what is going on. In either case, you want to call this to the attention of the physician. Don't generalize; tell the doctor only what you personally have experienced, not what others have told you. Don't speak for others. Be sure that you have observed this behavior more than once and that you are sure it is discourteous. Do it at the beginning of your next visit, with no staff persons present; if a staff member is present, politely say, "I need to talk privately with the doctor; will you please excuse us for a few minutes?"

Report your findings and feelings to the doctor politely and without anger. Do not attack the personalities or behavior of anyone in the office, but report it simply and say, "It makes me feel unwanted and uncomfortable."

If the doctor is negative to your complaints, or over-excuses them, or refuses to accept what you say, you will know that he doesn't care or else you are mistaken. Then your options are open.

If you stay, watch and see what happens on the next visit. If there is change, be sure to thank the doctor and say a nice word to the staff person or persons. That's called positive reinforcement.

If there is no change (and the physician has indicated that changes would be made), report it to the doctor one more time. No results? You now have options.

Always remember that you are the patient and someone is paying that office for your care. You are entitled to polite handling and courtesy by everyone and, if you do not get it, it is your option to leave for another doctor.

I see a different doctor or assistant each time I come to the office

There are philosophical differences among offices with more than one physician. Some feel that the individual is a patient of the "office" and that they can best render service by always having some physician there to see you. And, if you see several different doctors on different visits, you will almost always see a doctor who has seen you before and understands your case. But you should be told this arrangement on your first visit.

Some offices feel the same but try—the operative word is "try"—to have you see the same doctor whenever possible—if that doctor has hours when you want to come in and if the staff tries to make such arrangement.

Other "offices" assign you to a doctor and you will see that physician every time except possibly in an emergency. This essentially gives you your private physician who works in an office with other physicians who see other persons.

Take your choice of what you like. Ask on your first visit to a group about how they work. If you like it, stay. If you prefer another system, leave to go to an office more like what you want.

I want a second opinion, but I am afraid of hurting my doctor's feelings. I feel the need for referral to a specialist, but my doctor will not send me.

Most physicians would not object to recommending a consultation, as it protects him also. Since no one is perfect, it is always good to get a confirmation of a decision, or another opinion. Obviously, no patient should approach the subject by saying, "Doctor, I'm not satisfied with what you are doing and I want to see someone else."

Done properly, this should be smooth. "Doctor, I'm very concerned about this problem (diagnosis, treatment)." Then, "Doctor, could you recommend a consultant to see me?" Or, if you have already decided, "Doctor, would it be alright if I saw Dr. Jones in consultation—I understand he is very good at this sort of thing. I really want to keep you as my physician—but I just want another opinion."

Arrogance, defensiveness, refusal or similar such behavior tells you something about your doctor. Go see the consultant anyway. I believe the overwhelming majority of physicians would be glad to accommodate a patient's request for a second opinion; it will either confirm what your doctor said, or add another dimension to your care.

However, don't fail to ask for permission – and asking civilly.

What should a physical exam consist of?

The simple answer is that it should be complete enough to give the physician the information needed to make a diagnosis and to prescribe treatment. But that's not as simple as it sounds.

If your doctor takes a satisfactory history, he may already have a good idea where to look and how complete the physical exam should be.

For a first visit, it should really be complete. The physician must know your body –because all the parts of it are connected and inter-related. An otorhinolayngologist needs to ascertain your blood pressure before he can treat the ringing in your ears from his/her specialty standpoint. A dermatologist probably will want to see whether your nose and throat show signs of some allergy if you are complaining of an itchy skin rash. Most specialists will do a brief general screening (after taking your history) and then concentrate on the specialty area.

The more vague or generalized your complaint, the more intensive the physical examination will have to be. A problem of recurring headache, for example, demands consideration of a number of systems—cardiovascular, neurological, visual and others, so a more thorough examination is indicated.

Once again, it is your responsibility to speak up if you feel that you are not getting a complete enough examination. Ask why your blood pressure wasn't taken, or your ears looked at or your belly examined—if you think that part of the examination was important.

If your doctor takes an 11-second history of your problem and then looks at one thing (eyes, throat, belly, heart, etc.), you are not being examined properly no matter how confident the doctor is or how good his reputation is. Rare is the doctor who can do that successfully—and, thank goodness, very rare is the doctor who tries.

How and when should I learn results of tests?

If it is a routine test— for example, a thyroid function test that your doctor is just periodically checking – you can wait until your next visit. However, if your tests are urgent because you are searching for a diagnosis or treatment, or if a routine test is abnormal, you are entitled to a call from the doctor – not an aide—to tell you about it and explain its importance. Hopefully, he will do it in a kind and humane manner. A psychologist I know went for a breast biopsy. One night, two days later, the doctor called her and with no preliminaries, said, "Your biopsy shows cancer. I want you in the hospital tomorrow morning for surgery." Pretty crude. Pretty blunt. Pretty alarming. But not very pretty at all!

Once more, if the test is frightening or threatening to you, or you are worried about it, call your physicians a day or two after the test and start to ask questions—best if you speak to him/her and not an aide. It's **your** test. It's **your** life and health. Someone (you? me?) is paying for your test. There is an obligation to tell you the results—and in a timely manner.

I sometimes receive medications without an explanation of what they are for. When tests are ordered, I'm not always sure what they are for and if they are needed. I often feel out of control of my medical care.

All of the complaints listed here are related. They indicate that there is not complete or satisfactory communication between doctor and patient. Speak up or change doctors. In most instances, your physician will be happy to know how you feel about his care of you, pleased to know where he appears to be incomplete and glad to keep a patient satisfied.

If you want satisfactory care, if you want to be totally informed about your health, if you want not to be unhappy, ask questions and get satisfactory answers. **It is your responsibility to look after your own health and your responsibility to get adequate answers from your health care professional.** The overwhelming number of physicians would want this for you, and will cooperate with you in seeking the best care you can get. If your doctor doesn't fit this bill to your satisfaction, get one who does.

Remember that all doctors are different, even though there are parameters for proper behavior. One doctor, for example, may take your hand, or put an arm on your shoulder when telling you about a bad result. Another doctor may sit across the desk and in a totally "objective" manner, announce the results. Or anywhere in-between. Some patients prefer one type; some patients prefer the other.

First, you should choose the kind of personality you want your physician to have. Then you will not feel uncomfortable with what he or she does or how he or she behaves. If your needs and the doctor's behavior do not match, get another doctor. Both of you will be better off. But the responsibility is **yours.**

Another stumble spot — Hand-offs

One other situation that can lead to errors is called **hand-offs.** It is included here because most hand-offs take place between two physicians or among several physicians.

Hand-offs, it has been estimated, account for as much as 80% of serious medical errors, so special attention should be paid to this situation.

A hand-off is a transfer of patient care from one physician to another— whether in a hospital setting (very frequent) or as an out-patient. As understood by doctors, the transferring physician is responsible for communicating all pertinent data about the patient and the receiving hand-off physician is responsible for accepting and carefully noting all this material.

Problems can arise in many ways. Sender accidentally forgets one important piece of data or inadvertently mixes up some number on the data, or the receiver forgets to take note of (or write down) some important fact or data. Or something may have occurred between the time of sending and the receiving, for example, a newer laboratory result, a change in symptoms, alteration in medication being administered or many other such happenings. While relatively rare, it is an important enough risk for patient to be aware of it.

Here is an analogous example. Although not a hand-off, this consultation example makes this more understandable. A lady was admitted to the hospital for a non-related illness but her physician wanted a neurological consultation about the memory difficulties she was having. When the consultant came to see her, he looked at her chart. Within a minute or so, he said to the doctor sitting next to him at the chart desk, "Oh, this lady should have been on (he named a drug) a long time ago." Had he carefully examined the chart before spouting, he would have seen that she had been on that drug a long time ago with bad results. (In case you are wondering how this story got around, the doctor sitting next to the neurologist was a very close friend of the patient's family and reported it.) Just think, if this had been a hand-off, the neurologist, without thoroughly studying the chart, might have started that drug which previously had dire effects.

As a patient, you must not relaxedly believe that the second doctor automatically knows whatever the sending doctor knew because the second one has been sent that information. At the risk of annoyance on the part of the second physician, it is up to you to present all you know about your condition, its findings and any treatment so far administered. Insist on repeating it — for the sake of your own health.

TO PATIENTS:
YOU MUST TAKE RESPONSIBILITY
FOR YOUR OWN HEALTH CARE

CHAPTER FOUR

Pharmacists and Prescriptions

Many surveys in the past few years have reported that pharmacists are regarded by the public as the most trusted health professionals. Much of this is deserved.

However, several outside factors contribute to this. Pharmacies and pharmacists are much more standardized in their approach than other health professionals, understandably. Modern advances have reduced the number of prescriptions that have to be individually compounded by hand by the pharmacist, as in bygone years. This removes much of the individualism and variation that may have occurred years ago—with the greater possibility of error. The role of the pharmacist has shifted mostly to dispensing—correctly picking the product your doctor orders, giving you the proper amount of that medication, and providing accurate instructions (your doctor's and the pharmacist's). Most of the medication is manufactured by the pharmaceutical companies and comes to the pharmacist ready to dispense to you.

Don't lose sight of the training of your pharmacists. They are just as learned in the art of compounding (taking the raw ingredients and mixing them together to form the medication ordered by your physician) as they ever were. They know what ingredients are in every medication sold and how the medications were manufactured. And they have even more background and training that helps to serve and protect you. Pharmacists today are educated in clinical matters and often collaborate with physicians in many clinical settings. So pharmacists do not just count pills or pour liquid medication, they provide service and knowledge.

How do you choose a pharmacist? Like other health professionals, almost all pharmacists are competent. What, then, should you expect from your pharmacist?

- Courtesy, consideration, kindness and fairness, as with all health professionals.
- No inordinate delays in filling a prescription. Of course, there is always some time needed to do the work, even if there is no other person ahead of you.
- Explanation of how to take the medicine, what it is and what reactions might occur, unless you refuse this information. Many states have made this a requirement for all pharmacists and prescriptions, but occasional pharmacies do not do this adequately.
- Adequate answers to your questions about the medication, and even about your illness (to the extent the law allows). Ask your questions. That is part of the pharmacist's duties and responsibility to you. He may even, in problem situations, refer you back to your physician for clarification. That is not

evasion; the information you seek may truly be in the realm of the physician..

These parameters will help you to choose. Obviously, any pharmacist not providing these (and there are only very few do not do their job adequately) should not be patronized.

If you are in a new neighborhood, or if you are changing pharmacists, ask your neighbors (or friends nearby) to recommend. If they are satisfied, you probably will be satisfied. Consideration should also be given to the location and proximity of the pharmacy and your ability to get to the pharmacy – if you cannot get there, the pharmacy will not be much help.

The development of large national pharmacy chains has altered the outlook somewhat. By and large, you can expect the same kind of treatment and care in any single store of any large chain – exact dispensing, similar pricing and consideration for you, the patient. They have the added benefit of maintaining a nationwide computer record on you, your prescriptions, your allergies (if you reported them) and any incompatibilities of a new prescription with your present medication. But there are still hundreds of smaller (and small) individual pharmacies that provide top-notch professional prescription services. The key is in the pharmacists on duty, not the size of the store.

If you find a pharmacy that is convenient, fair in its dealings with you, satisfactory in price and service and staffed with pharmacists with whom you can have a pleasant and comfortable relationship (no matter what your neighbor says), you've got it! Stay there and not be swayed by advertising or "specials" as they relate to pharmaceuticals.

Cheaper cosmetics and fancier bottles of perfume should not be your determining factor.

Patient Responsibilities

Remember that you must take responsibility for your health care, and that includes prescriptions. It is your duty to check every step of the way on your pharmacist (and he wants you to do it). If you like your physician and you accept what he tells you, you are obligating yourself to see that every step after that is correct, that his orders and treatment are carried out fully and properly. Once your doctor writes a prescription (or calls it in), his area of overseeing your prescriptions is finished. The rest is up to you.

That means is that it is your function

- to check on what the pharmacist gives you
- check on the directions as given by your physician
- take the medication exactly as directed

To accomplish this, you must know exactly what drug the doctor has prescribed, how the doctor wants you to take it (how much, how often, how long, at what times). You should also know what your physician is treating you for, and what results he expects. He or the pharmacist should inform you of any side effects, or incompatibilities with your other medications or what allergies could occur. If there is any difference between what the doctor said and the pharmacist says, DON'T TAKE THE MEDICATION until you have discussed it with both of them. And, even after you start the medication, if anything seems different or foreign— such as taste, color, shape, size, STOP IMMEDIATELY and call your pharmacist or physician

Finally, you must observe and obey all special labels or instructions on the prescription—for example: "Do not take with food", or "Take with food" or "Take before meals" or "Take at bedtime", and so forth.

Risks

Once again, as with your physician, the risks with pharmacists and prescriptions are slim if your follow the rules. Even though rare, you should know them and be aware of the slim possibility; YOU ARE IN CHARGE.

Just how much risk is there, even though I've said it is minimal? MEDMARX is an anonymous, national reporting data base operated by the authoritative United States Pharmacopeia, and contributed to by about 500 health care centers and systems, including a large number of hospitals and health care systems. With millions of medications prescribed in that data base, MEDMARX documented in one year 105,603 errors; although it is a large number, it is a small percentage, probably less than one percent. Of those errors, the large majority were corrected before causing harm to the patient, and only 190 errors resulted in patient injury. That is a very small number, unless you or your child were one of the 190, then it was 100%. And these numbers represent large operations, not private physicians and other clinics throughout the United States.

Senior citizens are at particular risk simply because of numbers. Seniors average 6 to 10 prescriptions. Remember that as we grow older, starting with mid-life, we gradually take more and more medications. So the risk is always there — and perhaps increasing.

Risks may be divided into four types: Risks occurring because of your behavior as a patient or parent; risks that come from faulty communication between your physician and your pharmacist; risks due to pharmacist's error; and other types of risk.

Your behavior risks

- Failure to take (or administer to a child) the medication prescribed or failure to take it properly. This may be one of the biggest risks of all. It has been reported that nearly half of all medications are not taken as directed. Some 14 percent of prescriptions do not even get filled, while 13 percent are filled but never used. Twenty-nine percent are filled and used but the prescription is never finished. These faults mostly may result in under-dosing or overdosing, neither of which is adequate treatment. As described before, the medication, to be safe and effective, must be administered when prescribed, how prescribed and the full amount of the prescription must be taken, unless you are told otherwise. Giving the drug at the wrong time, giving it too often, giving it not often enough or stopping too soon are all bad. A good example is antibiotic for a diagnosed infection. In today's market, patients do not have to be told that, to cure an infection, continued use of the antibiotic is necessary. Physicians will usually prescribe a certain number of days of treatment;

stopping it before that (maybe because symptoms have diminished or ceased) will result in incomplete therapy and perhaps recurrence. On the other hand, taking it longer than the time prescribed, may result in developing resistant bacteria and recurrences.

- Patients occasionally take someone else's medication because they seem to have similar symptoms. Some patients may go back to leftover medication from a previous illness because of similarities. Both are dangerous and this is high risk! Drugs may lose or gain potency on standing for long periods, so discard your prescription when you have run the course the physician ordered. (Ask your pharmacist how to dispose of unused or outdated pharmaceuticals. Different classes of medication call for different disposal regimens.) Similar symptoms do not mean you need the same drug as your friend or the same amount of the drug. DON'T DO IT!

- When visiting other health professionals (dentist, podiatrist, etc.), patients often fail to tell them what illnesses are being treated or what medications they are taking. This is important because those professionals may use or prescribe conflicting drugs without being aware of what you are taking. It is wise for all patients, especially those on several medications, to maintain a current list of all their drugs – as a reminder to themselves and for use with other professionals when needed. Lists are particularly good when visiting every health professional, instead of depending on your memory.

- The chances of difficulty increase if you fail to get accurate directions from your physician and share them with the pharmacist, or if you do not share all information with your physician and pharmacist about your allergies, drug reactions or other medications you are taking (even over-the-counter products).

- Patients sometimes do things to medication not called for. Some people crush pills that should not be crushed, in order to make them easier to take. Others cut pills in half that should not be cut in half. Some parents may just estimate the amount of liquid medication given to a child or dilute it to get the child to take it. DO NOT MAKE ANY CHANGES WITHOUT DISCUSSING IT FIRST WITH YOUR PHARMACIST.

- Putting pills into a container different from the original one can create problems. You may confuse them with another pill and take the wrong ones. You may also lose the directions for those specific pills. A great mechanism for avoiding problems with multiple drugs is the use of a daily pill box, marked by day of week or one which even divides the day into portions. Using these, patients can sort out their medications for the week by using their lists, instead of wondering what to do each time medication is due.

- There is a high risk in taking old or expired prescriptions because the drug may have changed — strengthened or weakened — by time, or your condition may have changed (even though you may think you have the same symptoms). The same is true of the mistake people make in sometimes taking other people's prescriptions just because the symptoms seem the same or the diagnosis is similar to the other person.

- Patients frequently are taking — or start to take after beginning the prescription — over-the-counter medications, herbals, minerals or vitamins. Some of these products may interfere with your prescribed medication. Be certain to check in advance with your physician or pharmacist about taking additional products.

Faulty communication

- A mistake in the filling of the prescription can occur (even though it is extremely rare today) particularly if the physician's handwriting is difficult to read. A common error, for example, would be to accidentally substitute Volmax for Flomax. However, if you inform the pharmacist what your condition is or what the doctor said the medication is, this is highly unlikely to happen.
- Similar errors can happen, if the handwriting is not clear regarding directions or amounts—but this is even rarer, mainly because those directions are usually written directly in pharmaceutical language.

It should be noted that in the past when a prescription was not legible (or the pharmacist felt that the drug or dosage was not the recommended one), the pharmacist was obligated to talk directly with the doctor to confirm what was written; or if he thought there was an error in the choice of drug or the dosage, the pharmacist needs to call the doctor. Many times in the past, this sort of communication prevented serious mistakes in filling prescriptions. Today, there seem to be fewer and fewer such calls— mainly because of improvements in our systems, but in some infrequent cases, a physician has felt insulted by such calls, diminishing the pharmacist's desire to call.

A great boon today is the use of computer-generated prescriptions. There can be no mistaking the typed words (even bad spelling is eliminated as the drug names can be stored in the computer). Some large hospitals use an electronic system that decreases the number of "incidents"; many physicians are starting to convert their own records to such electronic systems.

Pharmacists' errors

- Misreading of drug name or directions by the pharmacist—this is very rare and often prescriptions are checked by more than one pharmacist for just such a purpose.
- A miscount in the number of pills (or capsules) dispensed. Every human being can make such an error, even though pharmacists rarely do, in counting out, say, 100 pills. An even rarer occurrence (but one which has been reported) is a dishonest pharmacist who can make a few cents by providing a few less pills than charged for. Probably

this will never happen to you, but check the count of all prescriptions when you get home.

If there is an error, call it to the pharmacist's attention immediately—he or she will want to know. If it recurs, change pharmacies.

[A more dastardly behavior has hit the papers recently: a pharmacist was arrested for profiteering by diluting chemotherapeutic agents for cancer patients, selling a half-dose for the price of a full dose—and doing it persistently so that many patients were inadequately treated. The high-standard profession of pharmacy is besmirched by this—and we can be grateful that it only happens once or twice in a lifetime. Of course, the offender was jailed.]

- Errors occur more frequently when medications have to be compounded or diluted, as there is so much more single human judgment involved compared, for example, to manufactured pills.

- Calculations involving decimal points in preparing prescriptions are another potential hazard, as wrong placement can change the administered dose by a factor of 10. Again, mistakes are rare but do occur. A year or so ago, at Seattle Children's Hospital, as reported by the news media, an experienced pediatric nurse mistakenly administered 1.4 grams of calcium chloride instead of 140 milligrams (0.14 grams— ten times the ordered dose) to a small child, who subsequently died. Her 24-year record of making no mistakes on the job did not help her; she committed suicide. So there are two victims in such cases—the patient and the person making the error.

Other types of risks

- Incompatibilities between the new prescription and your other medications. Usually, your doctor will catch this. The second line of defense is the pharmacist and since most pharmacists now use a computerized check-and-balance of your medication, this will light up the board, IF you are getting all your prescriptions at one location. Often, these reactions may occur when you take over-the-counter medications – especially herbs and other non-prescription items — without telling either you doctor or pharmacist. TELL THEM EVERYTHING!

- Abbreviations offer stumbling blocks. Health professionals have a shorthand method of communicating — abbreviations. For example, in notes, on prescriptions, or in communicating verbally, one might say BID (bis in die) which universally means *twice daily* (but it does have a couple other meanings). Or, the abbreviation *p.c.* might be written on a prescription, meaning *after meals*. Neil M. Davis, Professor Emeritus at Temple University School of Pharmacy, wrote a fascinating book titled "Medical Abbreviations' in which he shows how such shortcuts can lead to dangerous situations. Among his 45 specific examples, he cites a prescription written as "Lugol's Solution OD", meaning to give this iodine medication orally for hyperthyroidism <u>once daily</u> (OD). But OD also means *right eye* and a nurse put this iodine solution into the patient's right eye. More than just risk, it was horrendous.

Ten questions to ask

You must remember that it is your responsibility to understand each medication you take, what it is for and how it is to be taken. One way is proposed in "How to be Drug Smart", Consumer Guide #1 from the AARP (American Association of Retired Persons). It suggests a list of ten questions for each of us to ask our doctor or pharmacist or both when dealing with a new prescription:

> What's the name of the drug you're prescribing?
>
> Is a less expensive generic version of this drug available?
>
> How much will I be taking and how many times a day?
>
> What time of day is best to take the medication? Should it be taken with food or without?
>
> Does the medication need refrigeration?
>
> What side effects, if any, might I experience? What should I do if they occur?
>
> Is it safe to take this drug with other drugs or supplements? Can I drink alcohol while I am on this medication?
>
> What do I do if I miss a dose?

How long will I be taking this drug?
Do I need to finish the entire dosage you're
    prescribing for me? What do I do if I
    feel better before that?

These are all important questions and you should get the same answers from both your physician and your pharmacist. They may save you later grief.

Special Considerations for Older Patients

Aging patients require special consideration with regard to medications. Older folks often lose weight as they age and a "standard" dose of a medication may border on an overdose for the elderly. Often their metabolism is greatly decreased, which also interferes with a medicine's action, and can make it too "strong" for the patient.. Sometimes the differences will create more side effects. These factors make it difficult to determine dosages and often means that the physician must calculate the dosage for each individual drug and each time it is prescribed. The more manual calculations it takes, the greater the opportunity for error.

So be sure to remind the physician of your age (the age of getting older varies from person to person), and double-check with your pharmacist. This is one of the reasons for putting a patient's age on the prescription. And don't forget that some herbs, vitamins and other over-the-counter products may interfere with your prescriptions. Therefore, be sure to tell your health care professionals what else you are taking.

Special Considerations for Children

Why are children different? They come in a variety of weights and heights. They have varying patterns of physical development and varying metabolic activities. A five-year old child may weigh 30 pounds or may weigh 50 pounds. Different doses of medication? In some cases, yes.

Because of these obvious factors, medications for children are serious situations. Research in the applicability and dosages of medications for children has been quite limited for many years; even now, such research is still in its beginning stages. Some medications are not suitable for children. Most of those used must be diluted to an approximately correct dose for children. Mostly, what we have done is create approximate formulas for diluting drugs to administer to children – and they are not always accurate. This manual method has been found in controlled studies to be fraught with great danger (even in experienced hands). Incorrect dose calculations have been found to be the most frequent pediatric prescribing error. Studies show that deviations in calculation can be as high at 100%

When a physician or pharmacist calculates a dosage for a child, there is always the risk of misplacing a decimal point and creating havoc. Sometimes the medication only comes in pills, and of only one strength.

Everywhere, there is a potential danger in medicating children. The U.S Pharmacopeia, an independent authoritative body that deals with all aspects of pharmacy and medication, recently came up with a series of Parent Recommendations to Help Prevent Medication Errors in Children, and all parents should keep this list handy while their children are growing up. Many of these refer to hospitalized patients. But briefly, certain recommendations apply to parent's administration of medication.

- Be certain to apprise your healthcare provider of all medicines the child is taking and of all known allergies (the child should wear a MedicAlert bracelet at all times if there are any life-threatening ones).
- Be certain that the physician and pharmacist know the child's age and weight, so that the dosage is appropriate. And the diagnosis, if possible.
- Be certain that you are informed with verbal and written instructions (either by the physician or pharmacist or both) about the child's medications, common side-effects and adverse events that should be reported to the healthcare practitioner.
- Be certain to observe the child for any unusual behavior (such as difficulty in swallowing or breathing) after medication is administered.
- Be certain, if the medication is liquid, that you have been provided with and use an appropriate, standardized measuring device. Particular attention is needed in measuring liquid medicine because household droppers and household teaspoons vary a great deal and the child may get an inexact dose. If your pharmacist suggests purchasing a specific measuring spoon or dropper (usually not expensive), he is not trying to make an additional sale but wants to ensure proper dosing of your child.

The United States Phamacopeia also has issued a special Recommendation for Health Care Practitioners for Preventing Pediatric Errors. These, too, are directed at reducing some of the possible risks from prescriptions. They include basing dosages on the child's age and weight, considering frequency of dose, seeing that dosage preparations are done by a skilled professional (preferably a pharmacist), use of unit-dose containers when possible, advice on use of appropriate measuring devices, abbreviations checked and symbols used on prescriptions should be universally accepted or spelled out, doses measured in decimals should be thoroughly checked, and seeing that clear verbal and written instructions be given to parents or caretakers. (See also Chapter 6 for recommendations applicable to hospitals and institutions.)

Observing these recommendations will go a long way in reducing medication and prescription risks. Already beginning, or on the horizon, are systems to prevent prescribing errors. They include use of bar-coding systems which match patient against prescription, and color-coding to assist in instantaneous recognition of proper medication.

Canadian and Mexican imports

Patients constantly raise the question of importing their prescriptions from outside the United States. Probably the safest source would be from Canada or Mexico. Some medications are manufactured outside the United States and often imported here. On the other hand, many of the medications are manufactured in the United States (under FDA jurisdiction), shipped to Canada or Mexico and then re-imported for your use. Or, they may be manufactured in

Canada or Mexico by a factory of the same manufacturer. If you want to save money, you can think about ordering from these two countries. Even though it is the usual way it is done, be sure the medication you get will be in the original factory-sealed container – most exporters will not sell partial amounts. Hundreds of US citizens are now importing their prescriptions, in order save money. All things being equal – and leaving out any discussions of legality (and there are disputes about this) — importing these drugs is a boon to many people, dominant among them is much lower pricing. But it is each individual's decision after consideration of all factors. You should fully understand what you are doing, but if you are not aware of them, do not do it. You should discuss this with your physician first, and then determine what you want to do.

Actually, the legal question is in limbo. There are arguments on both sides whether it is illegal to order prescriptions from other countries. Congress and some states have been debating the issue, which is colored by other loyalties and geographic location. To my knowledge, no one has ever been prosecuted for importing medications for personal use, *whether or not it is actually illegal* – although some sources make threatening noises about this.

Two caveats: Delivery, which is by mail, can take up to 2 weeks for refills and 3 to 4 weeks for initial prescriptions. So ordering an original prescription when your need is immediate cannot be done, making foreign ordering an impossibility. Second, you cannot order small quantities and third, time will not permit ordering prescriptions for acute conditions, for example, cough, pneumonia, allergic reaction. Also, if you need 24 capsules for a specific acute situation, such as pneumonia, you cannot obtain them in short order because they could not get to you for immediate use.

Generic drugs

Disputes often rage about the propriety of asking for or accepting generic drugs. For the most part, generic drugs are the therapeutic equal of name brands (assured by the FDA), but may have different inactive ingredients. Sometimes they have a different taste. Sometimes a different color. Sometimes a different shape. And sometimes identical. But to conform to FDA rules, they must be therapeutically the same. To be certain, ask your physician or your pharmacist and get their opinion. I personally have no difficulty accepting generic medications in almost all instances.

Money-saving is the chief reason for generic drugs. They may run half the cost of brand names. And that is a great advantage for most people. However, recently AARP reported that some drug stores are marking up generic drugs at a higher rate than brands. While the cost of generic is still much lower, in some cases there seems to be an undue profiteering. For example, they found that generic Prozac (100 tablets) costs $223.99 at one chain pharmacy, and their wholesale cost was $4.90. The approximate cost for brand name was $300. The mark-up for generics seemed to be about double the mark-up for brand names. (As a comparison, at the same time, the Canadian price for name brand was about $135.)

TO PATIENTS:
YOU MUST TAKE RESPONSIBILITY
FOR YOUR OWN HEALTH CARE!

CHAPTER FIVE

Prescription Products

A distinguished professor at a major medical school started each introductory course in pharmacology with this simple but emphatic statement to his medical students: NO DRUG HAS JUST ONE EFFECT. Simple, yes. But very profound. And it probably can be classified as a major underlying principle in creating new drugs, manufacturing new drugs—and accounting for many thousands of drug reactions and great numbers of calamitous incidents.

You may well know, for example, that antihistamines are used to treat many allergic conditions, but a major side effect is dryness of the mucous membranes, especially in the nose. Thousands of people take aspirin for the relief of minor pains and it is mostly effective; it is a relatively safe medication but carries with it the possibility of irritation of the lining of the stomach and increase of bleeding time (especially if you are on a blood thinner). These generally are minor annoyances, but can develop into major medical problems. They are called side-effects, except when they cause major problems, when they become strong culprits.

That's why every product enclosure spells out almost every possible side-effect. That's why, in many cases, your physician warns you about the side-effects and what to do when they occur. That's why the pharmacist may also specifically mention their possibility.

Risks you bring on yourself

Some risks are incurred by actions or non-actions of the patient. They include:

- Failure to follow prescription instructions— frequency of administration (taking the medication too frequently or not frequently enough, failure to heed notices like "Take before meals" of "Take with food").
- Taking someone else's prescription because of similar symptoms.
- Taking medication beyond the expiration date.
- Not measuring liquid medication accurately. Again, patients must use a standard measuring device, such as standard teaspoon, tablespoon, dropper or other liquid measuring devices, as household items are not always accurate or consistent

Risks with serious consequences

Without finger-pointing or indicting anyone, let's note that there have been and still are a myriad of lawsuits against drug manufacturing companies, mainly because of undiscovered or unanticipated consequences. Some have resulted in withdrawal of the product from the market, some ended with large financial settlements. These are not because of the ordinarily minor side effects noted above, but for major reasons: serious side effects, deaths, additional medical problems. Here are just a few examples:

- A law firm that specializes in litigation against pharmaceutical companies not long ago published on the internet a listing about 300 "defective" drugs.
- Consumers and insurers brought a class action against certain drug manufacturers, claiming they covered up negative study results. A proposed settlement was for $4.5 million to settle 140 pending cases.
- Wyeth, a major drug company, reportedly has set aside $14 billion since 1997 for claims against its diet drugs.
- Pfizer, the world's largest manufacturer of medications, has 9,000 suits against it for a diabetes treatment drug.

Once again, these are not mentioned to frighten patients; just to prove that the risk exists. We are not indicting these or any other companies, but use these examples, out of many, to show what is out there. So, any untoward reactions on taking a medication should be immediately reported to your physician, pharmacist, the manufacturer or any authoritative body. That also emphasizes our suggestion — an imperative suggestion — of Be Alert, Know That Risks Exist and may happen to you. That is what is meant by

**YOU MUST TAKE RESPONSIBIITY
FOR YOUR OWN HEALTH CARE**

CHAPTER SIX

Hospitals

Once upon a time, people went to a hospital to die. Today, they go to live, for the most part.

The tremendous growth and development of American hospitals in the past fifty years plus all the modern medical and surgical advancements that occurred in them, made the hospitals strong contributors to the great health advances we enjoy today. Think about just a few of them—a very few out of many: joint replacement; intensive and immediate cardiac therapy saving so many more lives and allowing heart patients to go home after a few days instead of three to six weeks in a hospital bed; new and unique management of premature babies, with many more of them living and with fewer complications; laparoscopy and laparoscopic surgery that both eliminate more invasive procedure or offer less invasive procedures; and emergency medicine emerging as a specialty (and what about the immeasurable gains made by the development of our great 911 system getting patients acute care much faster?)

In spite of their great contributions to our survival and health, and in spite of all the benefits they offer us, it is still hospitals which present the most risks in the health care system. Why should this be? Why, with all the modern advances, does the hospital offer so much risk?

Problems occur in hospital settings primarily because of human error. People do make mistakes, not deliberately, and many times unavoidably. Remember that you in your doctor's office are dealing, most times, with one to five persons and most of them do not affect your health. When you take a prescription to the pharmacy, one to three persons may be involved with your medication. But in the hospital, any hospital, every hospital, innumerable people are involved with your care, even when you do not know it or even see them.

Let's take a hypothetical example, a blood count — a minor procedure but real — with slightly different protocols in different hospitals. Your doctor, in analyzing your condition, decides to order a blood count (he becomes person #1). He writes that order on the chart (correctly, we hope). Then a nurse or clerk (#2) transcribes that order to a laboratory request (correctly, we hope). Perhaps a courier (#3), or someone, picks up the slip and takes it to the laboratory. There, a clerk (#4) accepts it and records it some place. A phlebotomist or a technician (#5) picks up the slip (reads it correctly, we hope), goes to your room (the correct one, we hope) and draws your blood specimen. He/she labels it with your pertinent information (correctly, we hope) and places it in the collection basket. That basket is taken to the laboratory. Someone (#6) in the laboratory does the testing (correctly, we hope). The findings are entered (#7) on a report slip (correctly, we hope) and given to someone (#8)— perhaps a courier — to take back to the floor (the correct one, we hope). There, a clerk (#9) takes the slip and attaches it (#10) to your chart (the correct one, we hope). Some short-circuiting may occur with improved methods, but it always an involved procedure.

That relatively minor procedure, a blood count, infinitesimal in the course of a hospital's busy day, goes through a possible eight or more sets of hands. There is no room for error. For this simple process every handling must be perfect—not 80%, not 90% but 100%. An error on the part of any one person could totally destroy the objective: a blood count for you on which your diagnosis or treatment may depend. An error could produce over-treatment or insufficient treatment. And two or more errors will multiply the risks!

All this complexity is compounded by the number of different services involved: laboratory studies, radiology, medications, nursing care, medical procedures, surgical procedures, food services and transport of patients.

This frightening scenario, as complex as it is, is not meant to indict hospitals but is given so the reader will understand why so many things can go wrong in a hospital. It's a miracle, and not a small one, that so many millions of things go right in hospitals every day throughout the country. Hospital executives and administrators constantly seek administrative means to reduce the steps in all procedures and make everything safer for patients. After all, they are primarily interested in providing good service and doing everything to help the patient recover, and it is also strongly in their financial interest to do so—a small human error can sometimes cost a great deal of money at law.

Already electronic and computer programs are beginning to boost the progress in this.

So what can happen?

Answer: almost anything. I will not belabor the reader with a list of the piddling discomforts that happen to just about everybody who is hospitalized—food problems (cold, tasteless, incomplete, not delivered), being left on a gurney without an attendant for long periods of time, inappropriate delays in getting tests or procedures done, incomplete explanations of what is being done —an endless list. Many of these inconveniences are unavoidable, and the avoidable ones are human mistakes.

Rarely a week goes by without a big newspaper story about a major incident—damage, illness or death—that happens in a hospital, many times in some of the best in the country.

The much-publicized case of Betsy Lehman, a nationally-prominent and syndicated health columnist, shook up the medical world. A patient at Dana-Farber Institute (a world-renowned cancer center), she is reported to have been given four times the proper dose of chemotherapy for four consecutive days. This happened in spite of her expressing concerns by questioning the nurse because she felt that what the nurse was about to inject did not resemble previous injections. She objected and a Resident was called. He insisted that the nurse was right and the injection was given in spite of the fact that a pharmacist had questioned it at least once. She died.

Little publicized, another patient at the same hospital at the same time was given the same incorrect dose of chemotherapy, and suffered irreversible heart damage, even though she survived.

Readers will probably remember from a few years ago the case of the surgeon in a Tampa, Florida, hospital who removed the wrong leg in an amputation procedure – it garnered world-wide notoriety.

This was not the first—or last – wrong-site surgery. More often than we would like, there is a report in the media of a surgeon who removed the wrong breast from a woman. Validating the prevalence of wrong-site surgery, the American Academy of Orthopedic Surgeons, recognizing that the problem existed and trying to set parameters for prevention, formed a Task Force on Wrong Site Surgery and in 1997 produced a report of that committee along with recommendations for prevention.

In Los Angeles, a 16-month old girl, admitted for a cleft palate repair, died from of lack of oxygen because a misplaced breathing tube was inserted into her stomach instead of her lungs.

But these things do not happen just in the United States. Reports are filtering in from the United Kingdom and other places in the world.

In Glasgow, the Royal Hospital for Sick Children found that their five-year error rate was one for every 682 admissions, an unusual (and questionably) low rate but a number still too large for comfort. None of these patients died but 10% required extra treatment. More than 50% of the cases were intravenous treatments including feeding fluids and about a third were medication errors.

In another case in the U.S., a family physician saw a patient about 6 AM one Sunday with signs suggesting a possible coronary occlusion. Utilizing 911 service, he admitted the patient to a local hospital and called the attending cardiologist with the necessary information, including the patient's medications. Shortly after admission, a nurse came in with two pills for the patient. Curious, and knowing his own medications, he asked what the medication was. Aspirin! In spite of his being on Coumadin (an anticoagulant, a blood thinner)! The patent refused to take them. They could have killed him, so he waited for the attending cardiologist, who showed up at 11.30 PM—18 hours after being called!! And when the patient sarcastically asked the doctor, "How was your golf game?" the cardiologist replied "Very good". Self-indicting.

A community VIP was admitted to a celebrated community hospital for surgery—with all authorities notified of his presence. He did poorly after the surgery, and was placed on a respirator because he was deemed too weak to breathe on his own. After several days with assisted breathing, his outside attending physician examined the chart and found that this patient – on thyroid substance for many years— was not given that medication in the hospital. No wonder he couldn't breathe. None of his physicians noticed that the essential medication he should have been given was not prescribed.

These cases were culled from a long list of celebrated cases and unreported ones, some causing death or other horrible consequences, some just illustrations of the variety of medical errors that can occur. I did this not to scare the reader or indict anyone but to emphasize the potential problems—and the severity of many. In every one of the celebrated cases, a great flurry of activity (real not artificial) sprung up to try to prevent future events. They ranged from pure finger-pointing to punitive actions to new organizations dedicated to preventing medical or surgical errors.

But were these isolated cases? Of course not. The problem is widespread. And it continues but more and more official and authoritative attention is being paid to it and improvements have already started.

How extensive is the danger? What are the statistics?

An Institute of Medicine report (*To Err is Human*) in 2000 found that up to 98,000 Americans died in hospitals from medical mistakes, with over 1,000,000 injuries. Most of those are probably due to medication errors, the largest component of medical errors, and the rest are probably errors of the medical care system, especially hospital infections. In 2010, the U.S. Department of Health and Human Services reported that 1 in 7 Medicare patients experience serious harm because of medical and surgical errors, accounting for about 180,000 deaths — about double the 2000 estimate.

You may wonder what dangers and how much danger exists if you enter a hospital. There is no accurate measure of errors that do occur. Suffice it to say that almost anything can happen to almost anybody. All the more reason for each individual to keep track of his or her personal medical care — and to ask questions.

An article in a prestigious medical journal pointed out that errors caused an average 270 deaths a day, the same number of persons who would be on a fully-loaded 757 airplane. The economic cost to the country was estimated to be $17 to $29 billion every year. (Imagine a 757 plane crashing every single day—what an outcry would arise!)

Using national figures, a Massachusetts group tried to estimate what their morbidity and mortality figures meant to Massachusetts. Their conclusion: 230-461 hospital patients are seriously injured by mistakes each week. Looking at deaths, they extrapolated from the U.S. statistics that 24 to 50 people are killed each week by medical errors in Massachusetts. Caution—these are estimates, unreliable for accuracy, dependent on the hospital, the hospital size, the location and the mix of patients, BUT it does gives a good view of the seriousness of the problems of hospital errors.

The United States Pharmacopeia did a study in 2001 through its reporting base known as MEDMARX. (The USP is a highly-recognized non-governmental agency devoted to ensuring quality of medicines and other health care techniques.) They documented 105,603 errors in medication of which 3,361 (or 3.2%) involved children. They said that "although the vast majority of errors were corrected before causing harm to the patient, 190 errors or 5.7 percent of the total errors, resulted in patient injury." Of those injured, 156 had temporary injury and some intervention was required and 31 of the patents had to have some hospitalization including one who needed life support and two patients who died. A sacrifice of life and money.

'Nuf said! Further recitals of statistics—and there are hundreds more— only reinforce what everyone, both healthcare professionals and the lay public, already know: hospitals and medication are dangerous because of medical errors, many of which are preventable.

To repeat once more, none of these errors are intentional, most are human errors, but all of them cause problems.

Is anything being done?

Yes, there is. Will it solve the problems? In spite of improvements from the new programs, the problem remains. Probably most of the recommendations will help reduce the incidents. Is it enough? I don't think so.

There is activity everywhere. If we judge by previous crises in the health care industry, much of such activity will produce very little. However, there are many actions that if instituted would impact strongly on the dangers occurring in hospitals including medications.

A month after the teenager died in Duke University Medical Center, legislation was introduced into Congress to create a voluntary system for tracking medical errors, offering hospitals and doctors confidentiality. At the same time, this legislation contained the assurance that lawyers would not be privy to that information. If it's really important enough to enact such legislation, why is it not important enough to make it compulsory instead of voluntary? Do we want to save just some of the lives? Do we not want to walk on toes of the perpetrators? Do we fear them? The bill has merit but does not go far enough, and its future is questionable.

One promising recommendation, already instituted by some medical centers, is a supermarket-type barcode put at admission on the patient's wristband. In fact, the Food and Drug Administration has already indicated that it will require such a system. All prescriptions would be computer-calculated. Personnel administering medication would have to match the bar code on the prescription container to the patient's wristband. Any difference in the drug, the dosage, the frequency, allergic information or drug interaction would set off an alarm. Already, there have been reports, including information from the Veterans' Administration, of decreasing illnesses and reactions,.

However, before getting satisfied that these offer the solution to the problem, remember that, to work properly, these systems must be perfect— a formidable task. If the prescription is not ordered properly (wrong name of drug, wrong dose, wrong frequency), or not properly filled by the pharmacist, matching would not help. And, as always, computers can make mistakes (though not as many as the human), and can freeze, and can break down. (Remember the day the bank couldn't handle your transaction because the computer was down, or the airline couldn't book your ticket?)

And GIGO still applies: Garbage In, Garbage Out—so the entire system must be guarded very carefully. As good and as promising as they are, computers cannot guarantee perfection.

Another aid to reducing (or studying) medical errors was proposed by the FDA: compulsory reporting for *suspected* errors, to be reported within 15 days, instead of the present reporting only when errors cause serious injury. In addition, they want blood banks to report all *suspected* serious reactions to transfusions, instead of just fatalities as now.

Other legislation and regulation has also been instituted in many states. For example, Florida now has a law that prescriptions must be "legally printed or typed so as to be understood by the pharmacist filling the prescription; must contain the name of the prescribing practitioner, the name and strength of the drug prescribed, the quantity of the drug prescribed in both textual and numerical formats, and the directions for the use of the drug; it must be dated with the month written out in textual letters; and it must be signed by the prescribing practitioner on the day when issued." That means total legibility. It means the date is written as March 3, 2003, not 3/3/03, and the quantity written as "one hundred (100) tablets." This should go a long way to eliminating some of the errors. However, I know from personal experience that many physicians still do not adhere to these new rules. As a personal experiment I asked a couple of fine physicians of my acquaintance a year or so after the new Florida law became effective whether they were aware of it. When they both said they hadn't, I gave each of them a copy of the new law. A month or two later, I discovered that both were still writing prescriptions the same old way — actually flouting the new law. Habits are, by definition, well ingrained and difficult to break. So it takes more than strong regulations or laws to change bad habits.

The Dana Farber Cancer Institute, spurred by the death of Betsy A. Lehman, completely evaluated their systems and revised them. Other hospitals have been inspired by the progress. At Farber, oncologists no longer not write longhand notes. They use the computer with an electronic form, and only when that is satisfactorily completed, can the physician sign off. Even then, the orders go through a series of checks and balances. Conferences of physicians and nurses, patients and their families also meet to discuss ways of improving patient safety.

At their affiliated Brigham & Women's Hospital, using this system, the computer caught 400 errors a week out of 13,000 prescriptions. One may say that this is merely about 3%—a relatively small percentage — but it is significant for the 400 patients endangered. And deadly important if one of the 400 were you or me. A successful program for preventing errors!

The Cincinnati Children's Hospital has instituted a complete computer operation for its patient care. All chart entries are entered in the system, which uses both work stations and portable computers, eliminating virtually all physician handwriting. Built-in decision support includes all the needed ancillary information. An unexpected benefit that was found by using this system is the gain of 40 minutes on each shift by using the electronic system—that means almost an hour of additional patient care daily.

Also under development, and being used in a few trial places, is the personal digital assistant (PDA), which places all pertinent information from the hand-held mechanism at the bedside with immediate answers and controls, drug information, medical references and all patient data. A great advantage is that the PDA can be handed from shift to shift without leaving the bedside and, as they say, without losing a beat—and thus ensuring greater safety to the patient.

At the beginning of the century, there arose recommendations for a new medical position in hospitals — Patient Safety Officer—and ultimately, several organizations of this new breed were organized.

In 2002, one new national organization, the Patients Safety Officer Society, was set up to try to reduce preventable medical errors and enhance patient safety. Its work is just in early stages but by bringing together patient safety officers from throughout the country, and discussing what works and what doesn't, they offer prospects of improving conditions for patients.

One of the fascinating new projects, established by the federal Agency for Healthcare Research and Quality, has already shown marked results. Labeled Project RED (Re-Engineered Discharge), the AHRQ researchers worked on the problem that Medicare patients had a 30% readmission rate within one month of hospital discharge. Project RED devised an 11-point hospital discharge process for all Medicare patients. It was found to reduce the readmission rate by 30% and generated cost savings of $412 for each patient. A real double boost for patient safety. It has now been adopted widely, even for non-Medicare patients. And it taught us that many of our discharge instructions to patients leaving the hospital were faulty and did not accomplish what we intended them to do.

Let me emphasize that, while computer applications and system modifications will greatly improve patient care, they are mechanical and need to be treated with care. They cannot do the job alone; some human intervention and interpretation is needed. And adding human beings to the care equation tends to introduce additional risks.

Finally, let me re-emphasize the thrust of this book. Much of the activity described will lead to increased safety and decreased illness and accidents. However, the greatest safety precaution is the one you, the patient can take, by being alert to your entire medical care, and by speaking up whenever you have a question or concern.

From these new organizations, there arose bits and pieces of advice to help you help yourself. Warnings: First, not all of them are for everybody, and second, understand that you may often upset hospital staffs and physicians by your insistence on answers. Again, it is your life and you have a right to complete information before you put it on the line. On the other hand, most hospital administrations will be receptive to your need, to anything that may help them reduce errors—and help patients—and diminish possible lawsuits.

YOU MUST TAKE RESPONSIBIITY
FOR YOUR OWN HEALTH CARE

CHAPTER SEVEN

The Surgical Component

As mentioned before, newspapers around the globe reported on the case of a young boy in a Tampa, Florida, hospital a few years ago where surgeons, in an amputation procedure, removed the wrong leg.

Other recent reports included a case in Minnesota where doctors removed a healthy kidney from a cancer patient, leaving the diseased one intact, and California doctors who removed the appendix of the wrong patient.

Let me hasten to reassure patients that 95% of all surgical patients get through their operations without any mistakes being made. But that remaining 5% amounts to about 4000 such mistakes a year. Some of the mistakes are unavoidable, like certain unexpected infections or some special condition of the patient. But some are human errors.

Among those errors which should never have occurred is surgeons accidentally leaving a foreign object— towels, sponges, instruments — inside the patient, estimated to occur 39 times a week in the U.S. The average settlement for such cases is $127,159 — that's about $5 million dollars a week. Care at the operating table could reduce the problem.

Wrong-site surgery includes operating on the wrong site (right versus left, for example), operating on the wrong patient and operating on the wrong organ of the correct patient.

The Joint Commission, which accredits medical hospitals throughout the United States, has estimated that wrong-site surgery occurs about 40 times a week in the nation's hospitals

For a period of 20 years, a study showed that almost 10,000 malpractice claims for surgical errors cost $1.3 billion. One may say that such numbers are not great considering the number of surgical procedures done in the United States each year — and that's true. However, with avoidable surgical errors, one case is a 100% incidence for the patient affected. This can be an avoidable situation.

Citing additional statistics here — and there are a multitude of them — would only add to the truism that in any surgery, there is a risk.

The one bright light is that almost every professional organization — specialty groups, accrediting groups, governmental agencies — has started to study the problem and with new and strengthened recommendations they already have made some inroads into controlling it. And the studies continue.

Two major recommendations have been proposed by the Joint Commission, and where put into effect have already made an impact. This agency, along with many other groups, is advancing the idea of marking the surgeon's initials, with an indelible pen, at the spot where the surgery is to be done. Along with that has been the corollary to mark the opposite side (the knee or ankle or kidney) with a large NO. The second recommendation that seems to have some impact is the strong recommendation for each surgeon to do a "time-out", a conversation with the patient just before starting anesthesia or the surgery— and reconfirming what is going to be done. Already there are reports of decreasing incidence of errors from wrong-site surgery.

Wrong-site surgery is a major, major problem, but is not by far the only one. Every surgical procedure carries some risk, some major, some minor — even under the best conditions. Fortunately, the overwhelming number of surgical cases occur without error. But errors do persist.

For every one of the life-threatening incidents, there are hundreds of errors that do not result in death and go unnoticed or unreported because the results are not life-threatening or are minimal. A middle-aged gentleman needed a knee replacement. Wisely, he shopped around his community (and also outside his community), spoke to a number of friends and physicians and decided on a highly-recommended orthopedic surgeon. The surgery was done, but the results were not good. Only after he started to have difficulties, he learned — surreptitiously — that the surgeon he engaged did not do the surgery. A substitute surgeon had performed the operation, but the patient was never told, either before or after the surgery. Punch-line: The patient was a physician. If the original surgeon lied to a colleague, what . . . ?

But such recommendations or additional rules or other "policing' devices will not correct the problem alone. Each person, as I keep saying, must take responsibility for his or her own healthcare, because the only constant in the situation is the patient.

The federal Agency for Healthcare Research and Quality has issued a comprehensive "20 Tips to Help Prevent Medical Errors". The few suggestions to patients used here are derived mainly from that fact sheet.

What are some of the things the patient can do to take control of his own healthcare?

Check out your doctor and hospital. Certainly inquire about the number of cases (such as yours) the surgeon has done, and the hospital has done.

Wrong-site surgery. Has the hospital ever had a case of wrong-site surgery? When?

Talk to everyone at the hospital. Be sure all personnel know who you are and why you are having surgery.

Make sure your doctor, your surgeon and you all agree what is to be done.

Communication seems to be the keystone of prevention— talk between or among your doctor, surgeon, hospital staff, operating room crew. The more people who know why you are there, the safer you will probably be.

Talk to your surgeon about signing the surgical site or using other direct identification. But do not be put off with the occasional response of "Don't worry; we've been doing this for years with no problems." Your response might be, "But I am worried and I want some reassurance of my safety." A spotless record can be wiped out by one accident, error or misstep— even after years of work. Help prevent it!

All of this means that you—the patient, must keep as much control of the surgical situation as possible (or someone for you). Be alert. Be inquisitive. Be alive. And always remember:

YOU MUST TAKE RESPONSIBILITY
FOR YOUR OWN HEALTH CARE

CHAPTER EIGHT

Mental Health Care

First, a clarification: This chapter is not devoted to complications or risks of specific illnesses. That is for another work. For example, one of the risks of having a cold is the possibility of developing pneumonia — that is a risk of the illness itself. It is not the kind of risk to be reviewed here. On the other hand, the risks of *treatment* for a cold — such risks as covered in several previous chapters — are another story, like the theme of this book.

So this will not be a compilation of mental illnesses.

A confusing factor in the treatment of mental problems is the existence of divergence among different psychological or psychiatric "theories" and in the variously named disciplines— psychiatry, psychology, social work, counseling, and others, herein referred to as "therapist" or "prescriber" or "mental health professional". While all have their positives and negatives and there is frequently difference of opinion among them, there is generally a somewhat similar approach to these conditions. Some may use what patients call "talk therapy", others may not. However, one major separation of these disciplines is that <u>only</u> the psychiatrists, who are physicians — whether Doctors of Medicine (MD) or Doctors of Osteopathic Medicine (DO) — are licensed to prescribe medication. But like medical care in general, mental health care has its risks also.

Important difference

An important differential to me between medical care and mental health care is the importance of the family (and friends).While they are important in all care, being able to report what the mental health patient has not revealed may cast light on significant information for the mental health professional. The mentally-upset patient may have forgotten something important or does not accept it, or may not realize the changes in his or her behavior, or is ashamed or otherwise reluctant to tell it. Slight changes in behavior, new symptoms, new occurrences all may have major import. This information given to the mental health professional may aid greatly in the treatment, or, even more important, may presage more significant mental health problems.

The risks

All the risks listed in the first several chapters regarding medications, physician errors, pharmacy problems, pharmaceutical mistakes and institutional occurrences are just as applicable to mental health patients. One may be an out-patient (ambulatory) or a hospitalized patient, but the same risks apply.

Several ever-present risks must be considered with mental health patients:

Choosing the right therapist

There are some differences in philosophy among the many types of mental health professionals and sometimes those philosophies get in the way of successful treatment. There is no way to determine in advance which philosophy you should seek out. A warning: Avoid "therapists" who advertise. The safest thing to do is to seek and to follow the recommendation of your regular physician.

Probably the only reason for seeking a change in your therapist or looking for a therapist of another "school of mental health" is the failure of the patient to improve. If the decision is made to find another therapist when dissatisfied, seek help in making a new choice— your family physician or some other knowledgeable person. Do not guess!

Problems with medications

Psychotherapeutic drugs, like many other pharmaceuticals, are potent— and as such, may have many side effects So when they are being used, careful observation of the patient is important, both by the patient himself and by loved ones. Any changes in the patient, minor or major, medical or behavioral, should be reported immediately (unless the prescriber has given other instructions).

Weight Gain

This, too, is another risk in the treatment of mental health patients.

Weight gain may be due to certain medications or to the patient's indifference to matters of health. It may occur any time in patients' treatment, during either initial therapy or when in maintenance therapy.

Once again, this calls for mental health patients — or their families — to take responsibility and keep track of their weight, and report directly to the treating professional or therapist any increases in weight or suspicions of weight gain.

Suicide and Violence

Mental health patients, both those hospitalized and those being treated on the outside, but especially those who are in-patients, run a much higher rate of suicide than the general population. Recently discharged psychiatric patients may carry even a higher expectation of suicide or suicide attempts, but it may occur any time during patient's treatment. Some psychiatric patients, especially in-patients, may have suicide thoughts and may even try to act them out. Most therapists recognize this, but if the tell-tale signs are not obvious, the help of family and friends is important. Every symptom related to suicide, every suspicious word of conversation should be reported to the therapist, and promptly. What may sound like idle threats ("I think I'll kill myself," "I'll be better off dead") or any even mildly suggestive uttering, even said "as a joke" and with a smile or a laugh, must be taken seriously and promptly.

Violence — against self or others — may also occur in mental health patients, and may be voiced by the patient (as in threats or revenge). This, too, is an urgent situation and should be reported at once to the treating professional or to the institution.

Here is where the oft-repeated admonition in this book *You must take responsibility for your own health care* needs to be modified slightly. While it still is correct in psychiatric

Arnold Melnick, DO

disorders, it has special application for families. Those loved ones surrounding mental health patients need to be alert for any possible clues: verbalizations — even mention — of suicide, new changes in behavior, puzzling actions or talk— or any change that stirs the family, must be reported to the mental health professional— immediately. Do not wait for an "opportune" time.

YOU MUST TAKE RESPONSIBILITY FOR YOUR OWN HEALTH CARE (OR YOUR FAMILY SHOULD)

CHAPTER NINE

Patient-created Risks
(Families, Children and Schools)

Every day, every one of us, purposely or accidentally, does things that add to or create health risks for us. Simple illustrations would be not watching where we are walking thus tripping over something, lack of care crossing a street, eating something we are not sure is safe, or thousands of other human actions. Those are not for discussion here. Nor will this chapter try to name every possible human risk. Suffice it to say, this chapter will attempt to make readers conscious of some health risks that we encounter almost daily and which may expose us to health care risks.

A few examples presented here represent some typical actions. Some have been mentioned before but bear repetition.

Medication

Not following directions.

Any number of moves may create problems: not taking (or giving) medication on time, skipping doses, not measuring liquid medication accurately (e.g., household teaspoons vary greatly in their content, often being more or less than an accurate teaspoon amount) or not administering the full daily amount ("She falls asleep before her last dose" or "He fights me at lunch time").

Ending medication too soon.

Rationalizations may occur: "My symptoms have gone, why continue it" or "I have enough relief that I don't think I need to continue the medication". Some patients take the attitude that they do not have to continue the medication once they begin to feel better. Doctors usually prescribe the total amount of medication (number of pills or amount of liquid) that they believe is the amount the patient needs for the proper treatment of the condition. So unless the doctor has instructed you otherwise, stopping the medication early may create the risk of inadequate treatment and may lead to further problems.

Continuing medication or treatment too long.

Similarly, this may lead to other complications or to toxicity because of "overdose" of the medication. It is an incorrect attitude to believe that "if the medication or treatment is helpful in curing what I have, it couldn't hurt to take it a few more days to prevent a recurrence."

One of the most blatant situations regarding treatment I have encountered was a man who, while being treated for a foot fungus, was told to wear only white socks (so that they could be boiled clean). Years later, he was still wearing only white socks because he thought it was good for his feet.

Children

It is nearly impossible to catalogue all the health risks children face daily, especially in their normal routines of playing, swinging on swings. engaging in sports and a myriad of other activities. Fortunately, most lead to no problems, but the health risks are always there. And many of the health risks described in adults are often the same risks for children.

Two stand-outs are noted in children:

Allowing children to take their own medication.

No parent would try to let a very small child take his or her medication alone (without supervision). But sometime in the life of a child, a parent may entrust this serious business to the child, depending on the parent and the maturity of the child— 14? 16? 18?. No uniform age can be assumed. But it is always more prudent to wait until the child is older and more responsible — that is the safe way.

Children, medication and school. Many times, a child is on chronic medication but is healthy enough to attend school or is taking medication for a current condition that requires regular periodic administration. Then there arises the need to send the medication to school and ask the teacher to administer it, in order to keep the doctor-prescribed schedule.

The health care risks here demand the following considerations: Does the teacher have any experience handling medication? Or in giving medication to a child (especially liquids to younger kids)? Is there time enough for the teacher to be able to administer the medication in a timely fashion? Who will handle or hold on to the medication between doses? What is the attitude (or policy) of the school? And there are many other possibilities.

Fortunately, this happens many times in a school year with total safety. Many teachers are asked to do this, and they complete it satisfactorily. We do not consider that the teachers are not medical personnel nor do they have medical training, so we are putting a lot of responsibility into their hands. Even though most parents do this cavalierly, fortunately for all of us, the teachers are intelligent individuals, and respond beautifully. But now this is your child in his or her school with a specific teacher and you have a special concern.

In some instances a school nurse is available, and this can add to your security. When one is available, you should request that the nurse handle the medication.

But first, always ask your doctors what they think and how it should be handled. If it's going to be a long period of medication, it might be wise to personally confer with the nurse or teacher and point out any specific worries or dangers. Let the teacher know what events you should be immediately informed about.

Following the doctor's recommendations is the most important first step and then your keeping close supervision of the entire situation. This will help reduce risks. Again, it is most important to follow this rule:

**YOU MUST TAKE RESPONSIBILITTY
FOR YOUR OWN HEALTH CARE
(AND THAT INCLUDES YOUR
CHILD'S HEALTH CARE)**

CHAPTER TEN

A Look Ahead

Before we start our look ahead, it is imperative that we examine once more the salient points made at the beginning of this book:

> **There is almost nothing in life that is free of risk.**
>
> **Nothing in this book is used to "scare" readers, only to alert all patients to common possibilities.**
>
> **Not every possible risk is listed here— only a number of "fairly typical" examples.**

And our conclusion for all of the risks:

YOU MUST TAKE RESPONSIBILITY FOR YOUR OWN HEALTH CARE!

Throughout this book, there are references to multiple prestigious medical organizations (medical, governmental and hospital groups) that are concerned with risk problems. (See particularly Chapter 6 on Hospitals) They are all studying these risks constantly and have already produced requirements or suggestions which are on their way to reducing greatly — or eliminating — a number of these risks. And their work continues. So there is a bright light in the future!

It is my opinion that as the years progress, other organizations will take up the study of risk factors that are within their purview— and these, too, will reduce health care risks even further.

BUT, and there is always a "but", there are some risks and dangers that are beyond our knowledge or understanding or recognition, so it is almost impossible to eliminate <u>all</u> risks. So even with all the attention that we are paying to the problems, some accidents and errors will still happen, making our serious warning most important:

YOU MUST TAKE RESPONSIBILITY FOR YOUR OWN HEALTH CARE

The implication is that the patient or his/her family will be curious at every step of health care and will ask questions when things are not clear. Or when any doubts arise, they will seek responsible outside consultations for assistance in confirming or questioning anything that is bothersome. When requesting such outside consultation, one must seek an opinion from someone not in the same office or even the same hospital as the attending physician. This avoids conflicts of interest or self-protective offerings on the part of the advice givers.

When there is serious doubt (for whatever reasons) about any recommendation or procedure, unless there is immediate danger, the solution is "Wait" and seek additional advice. Never be railroaded into anything — without reasonable advice.

And it means being alert to every health care need and offering that may arise!

With the precautions offered, I wish all of you good health and good health care experiences, with as many risks reduced as possible.

We know that many risks are involved with health care, that your caution can prevent some of them from creating errors, and that you, the patient, are your own first line of defense, so at all times

YOU MUST TAKE RESPONSIBILITY
FOR YOUR OWN HEALTH CARE